Is She Into You? Decoding Her Signals and Signs of Interest

Chapter 1: Understanding Attraction

The Psychology of Interest

The Psychology of Interest

Interest in another person is a complex phenomenon rooted in psychological and emotional processes that shape human interaction. Understanding the psychology behind interest can empower men to navigate the often intricate social dynamics of dating, especially in the context of modern relationships. Factors such as attraction, compatibility, and emotional connection play pivotal roles in determining whether a woman is genuinely interested in pursuing a relationship. By recognizing these psychological underpinnings, men can better interpret signals and signs of interest, leading to more meaningful connections.

Attraction often begins with initial impressions, influenced by physical appearance and social demeanor. The psychology of interest suggests that these first encounters activate certain cognitive and emotional responses. For example, physical attraction can trigger dopamine release, creating feelings of pleasure and excitement. However, attraction is multifaceted; it also encompasses personality traits and shared values. Men should be observant of how a woman responds not just to physical traits but also to conversational depth and shared interests, as these elements contribute significantly to her overall interest.

Compatibility is another crucial factor in the psychology of interest. Research suggests that individuals are drawn to partners who mirror their values, lifestyles, and goals. This resonance fosters a sense of understanding and connection, making interactions more enjoyable and fulfilling. Men navigating dating should consider whether they and their potential partners share common interests, social circles, or life aspirations. When these elements align, it can significantly enhance mutual interest, making it more likely for a relationship to flourish.

Emotional connection is perhaps the most vital component of interest. This connection often develops when individuals share personal stories, vulnerabilities, and experiences. In contemporary dating, where superficial interactions can be common, establishing a genuine emotional bond is essential. Men should focus on creating environments where open communication can thrive, allowing for deeper conversations that reveal authenticity and sincerity. By fostering this emotional intimacy, men can gauge a woman's interest more accurately, as she will likely reciprocate by sharing her thoughts and feelings.

In conclusion, understanding the psychology of interest is essential for men seeking to decode the signs of attraction in women's behavior. By recognizing the interplay of attraction, compatibility, and emotional connection, men can navigate the complexities of dating with greater confidence. This knowledge not only aids in identifying genuine interest but also encourages the cultivation of deeper, more meaningful relationships. Ultimately, being attuned to these psychological factors can lead to more successful interactions, whether in online dating scenarios, age-diverse relationships, or any other context where connection is sought.

Common Misconceptions About Signals

In the realm of dating, particularly when it comes to interpreting signals from potential partners, misconceptions abound. Many men find themselves grappling with mixed messages, often misreading intentions due to preconceived notions or societal stereotypes. Understanding these common misconceptions is crucial for navigating the complexities of modern dating, especially in environments such as online platforms, where communication can be less direct and more prone to misinterpretation.

One prevalent misconception is that all signs of interest are overtly flirtatious or sexual. This belief can lead men to overlook subtler cues that indicate a woman's attraction. Signals such as sustained eye contact, genuine laughter, or engaged conversation can be just as telling as more explicit gestures. Recognizing that interest can manifest in various forms is essential for men seeking to understand whether a woman is genuinely interested or merely being friendly. This broader perspective allows for a more nuanced approach to dating, reducing the likelihood of misinterpretation and missed opportunities.

Another common misunderstanding is the idea that women are always indirect in expressing their feelings. While it is true that some may prefer a more subtle approach, many women are straightforward about their interest. This belief can cause men to second-guess themselves or misinterpret a woman's straightforwardness as disinterest. Cultivating the confidence to approach conversations with openness and clarity can help bridge this gap. By creating a safe space for honest communication, both parties can express their intentions more clearly, leading to healthier interactions.

Additionally, the notion that rejection is always a reflection of personal inadequacy is a damaging misconception. In the context of dating, a woman's lack of interest can stem from various factors unrelated to the man himself, such as her current life circumstances, emotional readiness, or past experiences. Recognizing that rejection is not a personal indictment but rather a normal part of the dating process can empower men to approach these situations with resilience. This mindset fosters a healthier outlook on dating, enabling them to move forward without the burden of self-doubt.

Lastly, the belief that age differences in relationships always lead to complications can be misleading. While it is important to acknowledge that dynamics may shift when partners are at different life stages, successful relationships can thrive despite such differences. Misunderstanding the potential for meaningful connections across age boundaries can lead men to dismiss opportunities with partners who might otherwise be a great match. By challenging these misconceptions, men can broaden their dating horizons and foster connections that are grounded in shared values and mutual respect, regardless of age.

In summary, addressing these common misconceptions about signals can significantly enhance a man's ability to navigate the dating landscape. By fostering an understanding that encompasses a variety of signals, embracing honesty in communication, reframing rejection, and recognizing the potential for successful age-diverse relationships, men can position themselves for more fulfilling interactions. Ultimately, decoding the signals of interest requires a balanced perspective that appreciates the complexity of human connections.

The Importance of Context

Understanding the nuances of romantic interest requires a keen awareness of context. Context encompasses the various circumstances surrounding a relationship, including cultural backgrounds, personal experiences, and situational factors that influence behavior. For men navigating the intricate landscape of dating, particularly in an era dominated by online interactions and diverse social dynamics, recognizing the importance of context can significantly enhance their ability to interpret signals and signs of interest from women. Failing to consider context may lead to misunderstandings and misinterpretations, causing frustration and missed opportunities.

In the realm of online dating, context becomes even more critical. Profiles can often present a curated version of individuals, where personal interests, intentions, and emotional availability are not fully disclosed. Men must be particularly vigilant for red flags that may arise from the way information is presented. For instance, a woman might express interests that seem inconsistent with her actual behavior or communication style. Understanding the context behind her profile—such as her recent life changes or previous dating experiences—can provide insight into her current emotional state and intentions. By approaching online interactions with a contextual mindset, men can better discern genuine interest from possible deception or superficiality.

Age differences in relationships add another layer of complexity to the interpretation of signals. Younger and older individuals often come with different cultural references, life experiences, and expectations regarding relationships. These differences can influence how interest is expressed and perceived. A younger woman may exhibit enthusiasm and spontaneity, while an older woman might demonstrate a more reserved or cautious approach. Context plays a vital role in bridging these generational gaps, as understanding the underlying reasons for differing communication styles can foster deeper connections and mutual respect. Recognizing that each individual brings their unique context to the relationship can help men navigate potential misunderstandings and appreciate the dynamics at play.

Moreover, building healthy boundaries in modern dating requires an appreciation of context as well. Each person has their own set of experiences that shape their comfort levels and expectations in relationships. A woman who has recently exited a tumultuous relationship may be more guarded and cautious, while another who is open to new experiences may express interest more freely. By understanding the contextual factors that influence a woman's behavior, men can approach dating with empathy and patience, allowing for a more authentic connection to develop. This awareness not only helps to establish boundaries but also encourages open communication, fostering a more respectful and understanding dynamic.

Ultimately, recognizing the importance of context can transform the dating experience from one filled with anxiety and uncertainty to one characterized by clarity and connection. Whether considering the nuances of international dating, the impact of emotional health on partner selection, or the balance between being single and being in a relationship, context serves as a guiding principle. By cultivating an understanding of the diverse factors that influence attraction and interest, men can navigate the complexities of modern dating with greater confidence and success. This deeper awareness not only enhances their ability to recognize signs of interest but also enriches their overall relational experiences, paving the way for more meaningful and lasting connections.

Chapter 2: Recognizing Signs of Interest: How to Tell if She's Into You

Verbal Cues

Verbal cues play a crucial role in the complex dynamics of attraction and interest in dating, serving as one of the most telling indicators of a woman's feelings towards a man. Whether you're navigating the world of online dating or engaging in real-life interactions, understanding these verbal signals can enhance your ability to gauge interest and respond appropriately. While non-verbal cues often steal the spotlight, the nuances of spoken language can reveal a wealth of information about how a woman perceives you and the potential for a deeper connection.

One of the first verbal cues to note is the tone and inflection of a woman's voice when she speaks to you. A warm, inviting tone often indicates comfort and interest, while a flat or disinterested tone may suggest the opposite. Pay attention to how she emphasizes certain words or phrases, as enthusiasm in her voice can signal genuine interest. Additionally, the frequency of her laughter during your conversations can be a strong indicator of attraction; laughter often signifies enjoyment and connection, suggesting that she appreciates your company.

The content of her conversation also provides valuable insights into her level of interest. If she frequently initiates discussions about personal topics, shares her dreams and aspirations, or asks you open-ended questions that encourage deeper dialogue, these are signs she is invested in getting to know you better. Conversely, if her contributions are limited to surface-level topics or if she seems distracted, it may be a red flag. A woman who is truly interested will likely engage with you in a manner that fosters intimacy and connection, revealing her willingness to explore a potential relationship.

Moreover, the use of playful banter and teasing can signal flirtation and interest. If she playfully challenges you or engages in light-hearted teasing, it often indicates that she feels comfortable and wants to create a special connection. However, it's important to differentiate between playful teasing and sarcasm, as the latter may indicate disinterest. Understanding the context and delivery of these exchanges can help you decipher her true intentions and reciprocate in a manner that fosters attraction.

Finally, consider the frequency and timing of her communication. An engaged woman will typically reach out consistently, whether through texts, phone calls, or social media interactions. If she initiates conversation often and responds promptly, it reflects her desire to maintain a connection. Conversely, sporadic communication or delayed responses may indicate a lack of genuine interest. By honing your ability to interpret these verbal cues, you can navigate the complexities of dating more effectively, ensuring that you are attuned to the signals she is sending and responding in ways that foster mutual attraction.

Non-Verbal Signals

Non-verbal signals play a crucial role in understanding the dynamics of attraction and interest, particularly in the context of dating. For men navigating the complexities of modern relationships, recognizing these signals can be the key to determining whether a woman is genuinely interested or simply being polite. In a world saturated with digital communication, where text messages often replace face-to-face interactions, the subtleties of body language, facial expressions, and spatial dynamics become even more significant. Non-verbal cues can provide insights that words may not convey, making it essential for men to develop their observational skills in dating scenarios.

Body language is perhaps the most telling form of non-verbal communication. When a woman leans in during a conversation, maintains eye contact, or mirrors your gestures, these are often positive indicators of interest. Conversely, crossed arms or a lack of eye contact may suggest disinterest or discomfort. Understanding these cues can help men gauge the level of engagement in their interactions, whether in casual encounters or more serious dating contexts. For those navigating online dating scams, recognizing the absence of these signals during video calls or chats can also serve as a red flag, indicating that the person on the other end may not be who they claim to be.

Facial expressions are another vital aspect of non-verbal communication. A genuine smile, especially one that reaches the eyes, can be a powerful indicator of attraction. In contrast, a forced smile or a lack of enthusiasm in facial expressions can suggest a lack of interest or emotional connection. Men should pay attention to these nuances, as they can reveal a woman's true feelings and intentions. In the context of age differences in relationships, understanding how facial expressions may vary across generations can also help men navigate emotional responses and expectations, fostering a more balanced dynamic.

Spatial dynamics, or the physical distance between individuals, can further illuminate interest levels. If a woman willingly reduces the space between you or finds opportunities for physical touch—like a light touch on the arm or shoulder—it typically indicates comfort and attraction. However, if she consistently maintains distance or steps back when you approach, this could signify reluctance or disinterest. For men building healthy boundaries in modern dating, recognizing and respecting personal space is essential, as it fosters mutual comfort and understanding in the relationship.

Finally, non-verbal signals extend beyond mere attraction; they also encompass emotional and physical health considerations in partner selection. A woman's non-verbal cues can reveal much about her emotional state, past experiences, and readiness for a relationship. Men should be mindful of the signs that indicate a potential partner's emotional availability, especially if they have children or are navigating complex personal histories. By attentively observing these non-verbal signals, men can make more informed decisions in their dating journeys, ultimately enhancing their chances of building meaningful and fulfilling relationships.

The Role of Digital Communication

The evolution of digital communication has transformed the landscape of dating and relationships, particularly for men navigating the complexities of modern romantic interactions. In the realm of online dating, platforms provide unprecedented access to potential partners, yet they also introduce unique challenges. Understanding how digital communication operates is essential for decoding signals and signs of interest. As men engage with women through various channels, the nuances of online interactions can significantly influence perceptions of attraction and compatibility.

One critical aspect of digital communication is the variety of platforms available, each with its own set of norms and expectations. Social media, dating apps, and instant messaging services all have distinct ways of facilitating interaction. Men must be adept at recognizing the subtleties of these mediums, such as the difference between a casual like on a post versus a thoughtful comment. Each interaction carries weight, and understanding the intent behind digital communication can help men gauge a woman's level of interest. Additionally, the immediacy of digital communication can create pressure to respond quickly, often leading to misinterpretations or assumptions that may not reflect true feelings.

Another vital consideration is the prevalence of online dating scams, which can distort genuine connections. Men should be vigilant about recognizing red flags that indicate insincerity. These might include overly generic profiles, requests for money, or inconsistent communication patterns. By developing a keen awareness of these warning signs, men can protect themselves from potential exploitation and focus their energy on building authentic relationships. This awareness not only enhances personal safety but also fosters a healthier approach to online dating, allowing for more meaningful connections to flourish.

Age differences in relationships are also magnified within the digital communication framework. The dynamics of attraction can vary significantly across generations, impacting how messages are interpreted and responded to.

Men should be cognizant of these differences, as what may seem like a clear sign of interest to one age group could be perceived differently by another. Effective communication requires an understanding of these generational nuances, enabling men to adapt their approach to better resonate with women of varying ages. This adaptability not only improves communication but also strengthens the foundation for potential relationships.

Ultimately, building healthy boundaries in digital communication is essential for fostering respect and understanding in modern dating. Clear communication about expectations can prevent misunderstandings and create a space where both partners feel comfortable expressing their interests and intentions. By establishing these boundaries, men can navigate the complexities of online dating with greater confidence, allowing them to focus on recognizing signs of interest and forming genuine connections. As digital communication continues to evolve, so too must the strategies employed by men seeking to decode the signals that indicate whether she is truly into them.

Chapter 3: Navigating Online Dating Scams: Red Flags for Men

Identifying Common Scams

Identifying common scams in the realm of dating, particularly online, is crucial for men of all ages as they navigate the complex landscape of modern relationships. As digital platforms become increasingly popular for meeting potential partners, the risk of encountering deceptive individuals rises significantly. Scams can take many forms, from financial fraud to emotional manipulation, and recognizing these red flags early can save both time and heartache. Understanding the common characteristics of these scams empowers men to approach dating with a critical eye, ensuring that they remain safe and focused on genuine connections.

One prevalent type of scam involves individuals who fabricate their identities to gain trust and elicit emotional responses. These scammers often present themselves as ideal partners, using flattering language and appealing photographs that may not represent their true selves. As men engage with potential matches, it's essential to look for inconsistencies in personal stories or details that seem too good to be true. A keen awareness of such discrepancies can help in identifying those who are not genuine and may be attempting to exploit emotional vulnerabilities for personal gain.

Another significant red flag is the rapid escalation of intimacy without a corresponding depth in the relationship. Scammers often seek to create a false sense of urgency, pushing for declarations of love or commitment in an unusually short time frame. This tactic is designed to manipulate emotions and foster dependency, making it easier for the scammer to request financial assistance or other favors. Men should be cautious of relationships that feel rushed or overly intense early on, as this may indicate ulterior motives rather than a healthy romantic development.

Financial scams can also be particularly harmful and often manifest when a supposed partner requests money under false pretenses. Common scenarios include claims of emergencies, travel costs, or medical expenses. The emotional appeal can be powerful, but it is critical to maintain a healthy skepticism. Men should ask themselves whether they have established a sufficient level of trust and familiarity before considering any financial assistance. Legitimate partners will understand the importance of financial boundaries and will not place undue pressure on someone to provide monetary support, especially in the early stages of a relationship.

In summary, identifying common scams requires a combination of vigilance and intuition. By being aware of the tactics employed by scammers, men can protect themselves from emotional and financial exploitation. This awareness not only fosters personal safety but also promotes healthier dating practices by encouraging genuine connections built on trust and mutual respect. As men seek to understand the signs of interest and navigate the complexities of relationships, recognizing these red flags can serve as a vital tool in their dating journey, ensuring they remain focused on authentic partnerships while avoiding the pitfalls of deceit.

The Psychology Behind Scammers

The phenomenon of online dating scams has gained significant attention in recent years, and understanding the psychology behind scammers is essential for anyone navigating the often treacherous waters of modern romance. Scammers typically exploit emotional vulnerabilities, leveraging psychological tactics to manipulate their victims. They often present themselves as ideal partners, using flattering language and deep emotional appeals to create a false sense of intimacy. This facade is designed to lower defenses and foster trust, making it easier for them to extract personal information or financial resources from their targets.

At the heart of a scammer's strategy is a profound understanding of human psychology, particularly the desire for connection and validation. Men, regardless of age, often seek relationships that provide emotional fulfillment and companionship. Scammers tap into these needs, presenting themselves as attentive and caring individuals who genuinely understand and appreciate their victims. By mirroring the desires and interests of their targets, they create an illusion of compatibility that can be difficult to resist, especially for those who may be feeling lonely or insecure in their dating lives.

Another significant psychological aspect of scamming is the use of urgency and fear. Scammers often create high-pressure situations, claiming that time is of the essence or that a dire circumstance requires immediate action. This tactic can trigger a fight-or-flight response, leading victims to act impulsively rather than rationally. Understanding this dynamic is crucial for men who may find themselves in similar situations. Recognizing the signs of manipulation can empower individuals to pause and evaluate the situation critically, rather than succumbing to emotional pressure.

Additionally, the impact of age differences in relationships can complicate the dynamics of scamming. Younger individuals may be more susceptible to the allure of romance and adventure, while older men might grapple with feelings of inadequacy or a fear of being alone.

Scammers often exploit these insecurities, tailoring their approaches to resonate with the specific vulnerabilities of their targets. By understanding the psychological factors at play, men can better navigate the complexities of online dating, making informed decisions that prioritize their emotional and financial well-being.

Ultimately, building healthy boundaries is essential in modern dating, particularly in the face of potential scams. Men must cultivate a sense of self-awareness and assertiveness, ensuring they remain grounded in their values and standards. Recognizing the red flags of manipulation and deceit is the first step toward protecting oneself from scammers. By fostering a strong sense of self and understanding the psychological tactics employed by scammers, men can navigate online dating with confidence and clarity, enhancing their chances of finding genuine connections while safeguarding their emotional and financial health.

Protecting Yourself While Dating Online

In the age of digital romance, online dating platforms have become a popular avenue for men seeking meaningful connections. However, while these platforms offer the potential for love and companionship, they also present significant risks. Protecting yourself while dating online is paramount, as the digital landscape is rife with scams, catfishing, and individuals whose intentions may not align with your own. To navigate this environment safely, it is essential to recognize red flags, establish healthy boundaries, and prioritize your emotional and physical well-being.

One of the first steps in safeguarding yourself is to be aware of common online dating scams. Many perpetrators disguise themselves as potential partners, often using fake profiles and stolen images to lure unsuspecting victims into emotional or financial traps. Look for signs such as reluctance to share personal information or meet in person, overly flattering messages that seem scripted, and requests for money or gifts. These red flags can help you discern genuine interest from manipulative behavior. Trust your instincts; if something feels off, it likely is.

Establishing healthy boundaries is another crucial aspect of online dating safety. Clearly define your comfort levels regarding communication, sharing personal information, and the pace at which you are willing to progress in a potential relationship. Communicate these boundaries early on, and be attentive to how the other person responds. A respectful partner will honor your limits and reciprocate with their own. This mutual understanding fosters a safe environment and encourages open dialogue, which is essential for any healthy relationship.

Emotional and physical health considerations should also be at the forefront of your online dating experience. Take the time to assess your own needs and desires before engaging with potential partners. Recognizing your emotional triggers and understanding what you want from a relationship can help filter out individuals who may not be a good fit. Additionally, prioritize your physical safety by arranging to meet in public places for the first few dates and informing a friend or family member about your plans. This approach not only protects you physically but also provides peace of mind as you explore new connections.

Lastly, be adaptable when it comes to the dynamics of online dating, especially considering age differences and cultural backgrounds. These factors can influence relationship dynamics significantly. Engaging with someone from a different generation or culture may require sensitivity and understanding. Embrace the opportunity to learn and grow from these interactions, while remaining vigilant about your own needs and boundaries. By fostering a mindset of respect and curiosity, you can enrich your dating experiences and develop more meaningful connections in the modern dating landscape.

Chapter 4: The Impact of Age Differences in Relationships: Finding the Right Balance

Understanding Age Dynamics

Age dynamics play a significant role in the dating landscape, influencing not only the attraction between partners but also the expectations and challenges they may face in a relationship. For men navigating the complexities of modern dating, particularly in the context of online dating, understanding these dynamics is crucial. The age differences that exist in romantic partnerships can lead to varying perspectives on life, communication styles, and relationship goals. Recognizing these differences allows men to approach potential partners with sensitivity and awareness, ultimately fostering healthier connections.

When examining the impact of age on romantic relationships, it is essential to consider the psychological and emotional maturity that often correlates with age. Younger individuals may prioritize excitement and spontaneity, while older partners might seek stability and long-term commitment. These varying priorities can create misunderstandings if not properly addressed. Men must be mindful of their own age-related expectations and how they align with those of their potential partners. This awareness can help in establishing a mutual understanding, ensuring that both parties are on the same page regarding their intentions and desires.

In the realm of online dating, where age discrepancies are increasingly common, men should also be vigilant about the red flags associated with certain age dynamics. Scams and deceit can disproportionately affect those who are younger or less experienced in the dating scene. Awareness of manipulative tactics that exploit age-related vulnerabilities is essential for protecting oneself. Whether it's a younger individual who may not have the life experience to recognize a scam or an older person navigating a digital landscape for the first time, understanding the risks associated with age disparities can empower men to make informed choices.

Building healthy boundaries becomes increasingly important when considering age dynamics in relationships. Men should establish what they are comfortable with regarding age differences and communicate these boundaries clearly. This includes discussing expectations about social activities, family involvement, and future aspirations. By fostering open dialogue, partners can negotiate their differences and find common ground, which is particularly crucial when one partner may be at a different stage in life. Healthy boundaries not only promote respect but also enhance the emotional well-being of both individuals involved.

Lastly, recognizing signs of interest can be influenced by age-related factors. Communication styles may differ significantly based on generational influences, impacting how attraction is expressed and interpreted. Men should be attentive to these nuances, as what may be considered a sign of interest by one age group might be overlooked by another. By developing an understanding of how age and generational experiences shape dating behaviors, men can better interpret signals and respond appropriately. Ultimately, understanding age dynamics is not just about recognizing differences; it is about embracing the unique perspectives that each partner brings to the relationship.

Societal Perceptions of Age Gaps

Societal perceptions of age gaps in romantic relationships can significantly influence the dynamics between partners, particularly in the context of dating for men of any age. Age differences often provoke a range of reactions, from acceptance to skepticism, which can affect how relationships are initiated and sustained. In the realm of online dating, where first impressions are paramount, understanding these perceptions is essential. Men must navigate not only their own feelings about age differences but also the societal narratives that accompany them.

Cultural norms play a substantial role in shaping opinions about age gaps. In many societies, there is a prevailing belief that older men should seek younger partners, while older women dating younger men may face scrutiny. This double standard can lead to discomfort for men who find themselves in relationships with significant age differences, especially if they feel pressured to conform to societal expectations. Additionally, the stigma surrounding age gaps can create challenges in how individuals perceive and react to one another, influencing the early stages of connection and attraction.

The impact of age differences extends beyond societal perceptions; it also encompasses emotional and physical health considerations. Men should be aware that partners of different ages may have varying life experiences, priorities, and health considerations. These differences can create both opportunities and challenges in a relationship. For instance, an older partner may possess greater emotional maturity, while a younger partner may bring vitality and a fresh perspective. Recognizing these dynamics is vital in building healthy boundaries and fostering a relationship based on mutual respect and understanding.

Navigating the complexities of age gaps also requires men to be attuned to the signs of interest from potential partners. Understanding how age may affect attraction and communication styles is crucial. Women of different ages may express interest in diverse ways, and men should be prepared to interpret these signals with sensitivity. Furthermore, awareness of red flags associated with online dating scams is particularly important in the context of age differences, as individuals may exploit societal perceptions for manipulative purposes.

Ultimately, the journey of navigating relationships with age gaps can lead to profound personal growth and fulfillment. Personal stories of dating success and failure illustrate that love knows no age limit, and emotional connections can flourish regardless of societal judgments. By embracing open-mindedness and cultivating resilience against external pressures, men can foster meaningful connections that transcend age. Understanding societal perceptions, acknowledging emotional and physical considerations, and recognizing the signs of interest will equip men to navigate the complexities of age-gap relationships with confidence and clarity.

Navigating Challenges and Opportunities

Navigating the landscape of modern dating presents a myriad of challenges and opportunities, particularly in a world where technology has transformed how we connect with potential partners. Men of all ages face unique hurdles, from the intricacies of online dating scams to understanding the nuances of emotional and physical health in partner selection. Recognizing these challenges is the first step toward turning them into opportunities for meaningful connections and enriching relationships. This subchapter will explore how to navigate these complexities while honing in on the signals and signs of interest from women.

Online dating has opened up a vast array of possibilities but has also introduced a variety of pitfalls, including scams that prey on unsuspecting individuals. Men must remain vigilant and informed about red flags, such as inconsistencies in a partner's story, requests for money, or overly eager behavior that seems too good to be true. By learning to recognize these warning signs, men can protect themselves from potential heartache and financial loss. Moreover, understanding how to distinguish genuine interest from deceit can empower men to pursue authentic connections, turning a potential minefield into a landscape rich with opportunities for genuine relationships.

Age differences in relationships can also present both challenges and opportunities. While societal norms may dictate certain expectations about age gaps, personal compatibility often transcends these barriers. Men must consider not only the implications of dating someone significantly younger or older but also the benefits that such relationships can offer, including diverse perspectives and life experiences. Finding the right balance requires open communication and a willingness to embrace the differences that may arise, ultimately leading to growth and deeper emotional connections.

Building healthy boundaries is another critical element in navigating modern dating. As men engage with potential partners, it is essential to establish and communicate personal boundaries early in the relationship. This fosters mutual respect and creates a foundation for healthy interactions. Likewise, recognizing when a woman shows signs of interest can help men gauge whether their boundaries align with hers. By developing an awareness of both their own needs and the signals being sent by women,

men can cultivate relationships that are not only fulfilling but also respectful and supportive.

In conclusion, the journey through dating—whether online or offline—requires a proactive approach to overcoming challenges and seizing opportunities. Men who understand the dynamics of dating, from recognizing the signs of interest to navigating the complexities of age differences and healthy boundaries, are better equipped to forge meaningful connections. Personal stories of success and failure can serve as invaluable lessons, guiding men in their pursuit of love while reminding them of the importance of emotional health and genuine connections. By embracing these principles, men can not only decode the signals women send but also foster relationships that enrich their lives.

Chapter 5: Building Healthy Boundaries in Modern Dating

The Importance of Boundaries

The concept of boundaries plays a pivotal role in the landscape of modern dating, especially as men navigate the complexities of romantic relationships. In the context of online dating, where interactions often occur through screens and profiles, the establishment of clear boundaries is essential for fostering healthy connections. Boundaries serve as protective measures that allow individuals to define their personal limits, ensuring that both emotional and physical interactions remain respectful and consensual. Understanding the importance of these boundaries can help men discern genuine interest from potential manipulation or deceit, thus empowering them to make informed decisions in their dating lives.

In the realm of online dating, where red flags can often be obscured by enticing profiles and charming messages, boundaries act as a safeguard against scams and emotional exploitation. Men should be acutely aware of their personal limits regarding communication frequency, sharing sensitive information, and the pace at which they develop relationships. Establishing these boundaries not only helps in identifying dishonest intentions but also reinforces self-respect and self-worth. A clear understanding of what one is willing to tolerate can serve as a powerful tool in recognizing when a potential partner's behavior crosses the line, allowing for a more mindful and secure dating experience.

Age differences in relationships further complicate the dynamics of boundary-setting. Men may find themselves attracted to women who are significantly older or younger, leading to varying expectations and life experiences. Establishing boundaries in these relationships is vital, as differing maturity levels can impact communication styles and emotional availability. Men should engage in open discussions about their needs and expectations, ensuring both partners feel valued and respected. This proactive approach not only helps in bridging generational gaps but also fosters a deeper emotional connection, ultimately enhancing the relationship's longevity.

Building healthy boundaries is equally crucial when considering the implications of dating single parents. When entering a relationship with someone who has children, men must navigate the complexities of blending their lives with those of the children involved. Clear boundaries regarding parenting roles, involvement in the children's lives, and the pace of the relationship are essential for creating a harmonious environment. By establishing these boundaries early on, men can demonstrate their commitment while also respecting the needs of the family unit, ultimately leading to a more balanced and fulfilling partnership.

In conclusion, the importance of boundaries in dating cannot be overstated. For men of any age, understanding and implementing personal limits is a fundamental aspect of developing healthy, respectful relationships. Whether navigating online dating scams, managing age differences, or engaging with single parents, boundaries serve as a framework for ensuring that both partners feel safe and valued. By recognizing the significance of these boundaries, men can enhance their dating experiences, cultivate deeper connections, and ultimately find the relationships that align with their values and aspirations.

Communicating Your Needs

Communicating your needs in a dating context is essential for establishing a healthy and fulfilling relationship. In the realm of modern dating, where interactions often occur online and expectations can vary widely, it becomes even more crucial to articulate what you are looking for in a partner. This subchapter will explore effective strategies for expressing your needs, ensuring that both you and your potential partner are on the same page as you navigate the complexities of dating in today's world.

The first step in communicating your needs is self-awareness. Before engaging with potential partners, take the time to reflect on what you want from a relationship. Consider aspects such as emotional support, physical intimacy, and lifestyle compatibility. Understanding your own desires and boundaries will not only empower you to communicate them clearly but also help you avoid situations that may lead to frustration or disappointment. This self-reflection is particularly important for men of varying ages, as life experiences and relationship goals can differ significantly.

Once you have a clear understanding of your needs, the next step is to express them openly and honestly. When dating, especially in the early stages, it is vital to foster an environment of transparency. Engage in conversations that invite your partner to share her expectations as well. For example, discussing long-term goals, relationship dynamics, and boundaries can provide insights into whether both parties are aligned. This is crucial in navigating challenges such as age differences or the nuances of dating single parents, where differing expectations can lead to misunderstandings if not addressed early on.

Building healthy boundaries is an integral part of effective communication. Establishing what is acceptable and what is not sets the foundation for mutual respect and understanding. This is particularly relevant in the context of online dating, where red flags can often be overlooked due to the excitement of new connections. By clearly communicating your boundaries, you not only protect your emotional well-being but also encourage your partner to express her own needs, fostering a reciprocal dialogue that can strengthen the relationship.

Finally, it is essential to remain adaptable and open to feedback. As relationships evolve, so too may your needs and those of your partner. Regularly checking in with each other about feelings and expectations helps ensure that both parties are satisfied and engaged. This ongoing communication can also help mitigate potential conflicts, especially when navigating emotional or physical health considerations in partner selection. By prioritizing open dialogue about your needs, you create a supportive environment where both partners can thrive, ultimately leading to a more enriching dating experience.

Recognizing and Respecting Limits

In the realm of modern dating, recognizing and respecting limits is paramount to fostering healthy relationships. This principle applies not only to personal boundaries but also to the dynamics of affection and interest. For men navigating the complexities of dating—

particularly in online spaces where signals can be misinterpreted—understanding these limits can mean the difference between a meaningful connection and a potentially harmful situation. Whether you're dealing with age differences, single parents, or cultural variances, awareness of boundaries is essential to ensure that both parties feel safe and valued.

One key aspect of recognizing limits is being attuned to verbal and non-verbal cues that indicate comfort or discomfort. For instance, if a woman expresses hesitation about meeting in person or sharing personal information, these signals should be respected without pressure or persuasion. This respect not only builds trust but also demonstrates maturity and emotional intelligence. Being able to read these signals is crucial, especially in the context of online dating, where profiles may project a curated image that doesn't fully represent a person's feelings or intentions.

When considering the impact of age differences, it's important to acknowledge that different life stages can influence comfort levels in relationships. Younger individuals may be more open to exploring new experiences, while older partners might prioritize stability and emotional security. Recognizing these differing perspectives allows men to navigate conversations and interactions with sensitivity, ensuring that both partners feel heard and understood. Healthy boundaries in such relationships are foundational to mutual respect and can help avoid misunderstandings that often arise from generational gaps.

In addition to personal boundaries, men should also consider the broader implications of dating single parents. These individuals often juggle multiple responsibilities, which can limit their availability and emotional bandwidth. Understanding this context is crucial for fostering a supportive relationship. It requires patience and flexibility, as the dynamics of parenting can affect how much time and energy is dedicated to a budding romance. By recognizing and respecting the limits that come with such situations, men can create a more accommodating environment that respects the needs of both partners.

Ultimately, recognizing and respecting limits is about creating a balanced approach to dating. It involves open communication, active listening, and an awareness of both partners' emotional and physical health needs. Men should strive to engage in conversations that clarify boundaries while being receptive to feedback. This practice not only enhances the likelihood of a successful relationship but also cultivates a culture of respect and understanding. In a world where the dynamics of dating can often feel overwhelming, a commitment to recognizing and respecting limits can pave the way for deeper connections and lasting partnerships.

Chapter 6: The Pros and Cons of Dating Single Parents: What to Consider

Understanding the Unique Challenges

Understanding the unique challenges in modern dating is crucial for men of all ages as they navigate the complex landscape of romantic relationships. With the advent of technology and shifting societal norms, men often encounter a variety of hurdles that can complicate their pursuit of genuine connections. These challenges can range from deciphering mixed signals in communication to grappling with the emotional intricacies that stem from age differences and varying cultural backgrounds. Recognizing these obstacles is the first step toward building healthier relationships and fostering meaningful interactions.

One of the most prominent challenges is the prevalence of online dating scams, which have become increasingly sophisticated. Men must remain vigilant against red flags that indicate deception, such as profiles that seem too good to be true, requests for money, or vague personal histories. Awareness of these scams not only protects emotional investment but also helps prevent significant financial loss. Understanding the tactics employed by scammers can empower men to approach online dating with a critical eye, ensuring that their search for companionship is grounded in authenticity.

Additionally, age differences in relationships can present unique dynamics that require careful navigation. While cross-generational relationships can offer rich experiences and perspectives, they also come with inherent challenges, such as differing life stages, values, and expectations. Men need to consider how these factors influence compatibility and communication. Finding the right balance involves open discussions about each partner's desires and concerns, ensuring that both individuals feel valued and understood in the relationship.

Building healthy boundaries is another essential aspect of modern dating that men must prioritize. With the blurred lines often seen in contemporary interactions, it's vital to establish clear expectations around emotional and physical intimacy. Healthy boundaries not only protect individual well-being but also foster respect and trust between partners. Men who communicate their needs effectively and encourage their partners to do the same create a safe space for vulnerability and growth, which is fundamental to lasting connections.

Finally, recognizing signs of interest can be particularly challenging in a world filled with distractions and mixed messages. Men should be attuned to both verbal and non-verbal cues that indicate mutual attraction. This awareness extends to understanding the emotional and physical health considerations that influence partner selection, as well as the implications of dating single parents or exploring international relationships with cultural differences. By embracing these complexities and remaining open to learning from personal experiences, men can enhance their dating journey, navigating its ups and downs with greater confidence and clarity.

The Benefits of Dating a Single Parent

In the intricate landscape of modern dating, single parents often represent a unique and rewarding opportunity for men seeking meaningful connections. Dating a single parent can be an enriching experience that offers a range of benefits, from emotional maturity to a heightened sense of responsibility. Understanding these advantages can not only enhance your dating life but also lead to deeper, more fulfilling relationships.

One of the primary benefits of dating a single parent is their emotional maturity. Having navigated the challenges of parenting, single parents often possess a level of resilience and self-awareness that can be attractive traits in a partner. They have likely faced significant life challenges, which fosters a more profound understanding of relationships and commitment. This maturity can lead to healthier communication styles, as they are typically more adept at discussing feelings and resolving conflicts, essential skills in any relationship.

Additionally, dating a single parent often provides a unique perspective on life and relationships. These individuals tend to prioritize their time and relationships, having learned to balance the demands of parenthood with personal interests and social connections. This ability to prioritize can lead to more intentional and meaningful interactions. Men often find that single parents are more appreciative of the time spent together, creating a shared sense of quality in the relationship that can be refreshing compared to more casual dating scenarios.

Another significant advantage is the insight that single parents bring into the concept of partnership. They are usually clear about what they want and expect from a relationship, having already navigated the complexities of previous partnerships. This clarity can simplify the dating process, allowing both partners to establish boundaries and goals more quickly. Moreover, single parents are often looking for a supportive partner rather than someone to fill a void, which can lead to healthier relationship dynamics and mutual growth.

While it is essential to acknowledge the potential challenges of dating a single parent, such as the complexities of integrating into their family life, the rewards often outweigh these concerns. Engaging with a single parent can foster a sense of compassion and understanding, as both partners navigate the intricacies of their lives together. This relationship dynamic can create a strong foundation built on mutual respect and shared experiences, ultimately leading to a more profound and fulfilling partnership.

In conclusion, dating a single parent can be a gateway to discovering the richness of emotional depth, intentionality, and growth in relationships. As men navigate the intricacies of modern dating, understanding the unique benefits of connecting with single parents can enhance their experiences and foster deeper emotional connections. Embracing this opportunity not only broadens one's perspective on love and partnership but also enriches the journey of finding a compatible and committed partner.

Strategies for Building a Blended Family

Building a blended family can be a rewarding yet challenging endeavor for men entering relationships with single parents. As you navigate the complexities of dating someone with children, it is crucial to adopt strategies that foster harmony, understanding, and respect among all family members. This subchapter will explore key strategies that can help you successfully integrate into a blended family dynamic, ensuring that both romantic and familial relationships flourish.

One of the most important strategies is to establish open and honest communication with your partner and her children. This involves creating an environment where feelings and concerns can be shared without fear of judgment. Discuss expectations, boundaries, and roles within the family structure to minimize misunderstandings. For instance, clarify how parenting responsibilities will be shared and decide on rules that apply to everyone in the household. Open communication also allows you to gain insight into the children's perspectives, helping them feel valued and heard as you step into their lives.

Building trust is another essential strategy when integrating into a blended family. Trust takes time to develop, especially with children who may feel apprehensive about new relationships. It is vital to approach this process with patience and consistency. Show up for family activities, be present during important events, and demonstrate reliability in your commitments.

By being a stable figure in their lives, you can gradually earn their trust and respect, which will facilitate smoother interactions and create a stronger family bond.

Equally important is the need to respect the existing family dynamics and the role of the children's biological parent. Acknowledging the relationship that your partner has with her children, as well as any feelings of loyalty they may have towards their other parent, can pave the way for a healthier integration process. Avoid attempting to replace the biological parent; instead, focus on building your own unique relationship with the children. This not only helps in maintaining the children's emotional stability but also demonstrates your commitment to supporting their existing connections.

Flexibility is crucial in adapting to the ever-evolving nature of a blended family. Recognize that challenges will arise, and the dynamics may shift over time. Be prepared to pivot your strategies as needed and remain open to feedback from both your partner and her children. Adaptability allows you to address concerns as they arise, ensuring that everyone feels included and respected in the family unit. Additionally, celebrating milestones and achievements together can reinforce the sense of belonging and unity among family members.

Lastly, prioritize quality time as a family to strengthen your bonds. Engage in activities that everyone enjoys, whether it's game nights, outdoor adventures, or simply sharing meals together. These shared experiences create lasting memories and foster positive emotional connections. By building a foundation of shared joy, you can cultivate a sense of belonging that bridges the gaps between family members. As you navigate the complexities of building a blended family, remember that the ultimate goal is to create an environment where love, respect, and understanding prevail.

Chapter 7: Emotional and Physical Health Considerations in Partner Selection

Assessing Compatibility

Assessing Compatibility

In the realm of modern dating, especially within the context of online interactions, assessing compatibility has become a critical skill for men seeking meaningful relationships. Compatibility extends beyond shared interests; it encompasses values, life goals, and emotional alignment. Recognizing these aspects early in the dating process can help avoid potential heartache and ensure that both partners are on a similar path. Whether navigating the complexities of age differences or the intricacies of cultural diversity, understanding compatibility is essential for establishing a solid foundation in any relationship.

The impact of age differences in relationships cannot be understated, as they often influence perspectives on life, stability, and future aspirations. While age can bring maturity and experience, it can also lead to divergent expectations. Therefore, assessing compatibility involves open discussions about long-term goals, family planning, and lifestyle choices. Establishing whether both partners are looking for the same type of relationship, whether casual or committed, is crucial to avoid misunderstandings that could arise from differing expectations based on age.

Building healthy boundaries is another vital component of assessing compatibility. In the digital dating landscape, where personal interactions can sometimes feel superficial, it's essential to communicate openly about individual comfort levels and relationship needs. Men should be attuned to signs that indicate a partner's willingness to establish boundaries, as well as their own readiness to respect them. This mutual respect lays the groundwork for a relationship built on trust and understanding, which are cornerstones of genuine compatibility.

As men navigate the dating scene, particularly when considering partners who may be single parents or hail from different cultural backgrounds, it is essential to weigh the pros and cons of these dynamics. Single parents often bring a wealth of life experience and resilience, but they also come with unique challenges, including time constraints and complex family dynamics. Cultural differences can enrich a relationship but may also introduce misunderstandings. Assessing compatibility in these contexts means being proactive in addressing potential obstacles and embracing the learning opportunities that arise from diverse backgrounds.

Lastly, emotional and physical health considerations play a significant role in compatibility. Understanding one's own emotional landscape and recognizing the importance of mental well-being can enhance relationship dynamics. Men should also be aware of the importance of physical health in fostering a long-lasting partnership. Compatibility is not merely about finding someone who shares your interests but also about ensuring that both partners can support each other's growth, health, and happiness. By taking the time to assess these multifaceted dimensions of compatibility, men can better position themselves for fulfilling and enduring relationships.

The Role of Mental Health

The role of mental health in dating and relationships is an essential aspect that often goes unnoticed. For men navigating the complexities of modern romance, understanding mental health is crucial not only for personal well-being but also for fostering healthy connections with potential partners. Mental health influences how individuals perceive themselves and others, impacting their ability to recognize signs of interest and respond appropriately. A solid grasp of one's mental state can enhance emotional intelligence, enabling men to engage more effectively in the dating landscape.

In the context of online dating, mental health can significantly affect one's resilience against scams and manipulative behaviors. Many men, especially those who are newer to online dating platforms, can fall prey to individuals who exploit emotional vulnerabilities. Recognizing the psychological signs of manipulation—such as excessive flattery, urgency, or inconsistent communication—requires a keen awareness of one's mental health. Establishing healthy boundaries is a vital strategy to protect against these red flags, ensuring that men prioritize their emotional safety while remaining open to genuine connections.

Age differences in relationships also present unique mental health considerations. Men dating younger or older partners may encounter different expectations and communication styles, which can create stress or misunderstandings. Being aware of these dynamics and maintaining open dialogues about feelings and experiences can mitigate potential conflicts. Acknowledging the mental health implications of these relationships helps men navigate them with greater empathy and understanding, fostering a connection that transcends age-related challenges.

Furthermore, emotional and physical health should be considered in partner selection. A partner's mental health status can impact the dynamics of the relationship, influencing everything from communication patterns to conflict resolution. Men should be mindful of their own emotional health and the health of potential partners, recognizing that mental wellness can significantly affect relationship satisfaction. Prioritizing emotional compatibility can lead to more fulfilling relationships, where both partners support each other's growth and well-being.

Finally, exploring the benefits of being single versus being in a relationship underscores the critical role of mental health in personal choices. While relationships can offer companionship and support, being single allows for self-exploration and mental wellness without the added pressures of a partnership. Men should reflect on their mental health needs when considering these options, weighing the pros and cons to determine what aligns best with their emotional well-being. Ultimately, understanding the role of mental health in dating can empower men to make informed decisions, leading to healthier and more satisfying romantic experiences.

Prioritizing Physical Well-Being

Prioritizing physical well-being is an essential component of building healthy relationships, particularly in the context of modern dating. For men navigating the complexities of online dating and interpersonal connections, maintaining good physical health can not only enhance personal confidence but also impact how potential partners perceive them. In an age where first impressions are often made through photographs and profile descriptions, being physically fit and healthy can serve as an attractive quality. Men should recognize that investing in their physical well-being is not merely about aesthetics; it is a holistic approach encompassing mental, emotional, and physical health that ultimately enriches dating experiences.

Engaging in regular exercise, maintaining a balanced diet, and ensuring adequate sleep are fundamental to physical well-being. When men prioritize these aspects of health, they not only improve their own quality of life but also display a level of self-respect and discipline that can be appealing to potential partners. Furthermore, physical activity has been shown to release endorphins, which boost mood and reduce stress. This emotional stability can be particularly important in the context of dating, as it allows men to approach relationships with a clear mind and positive outlook, making them more approachable and enjoyable companions.

Moreover, physical well-being can enhance emotional intelligence, an often-overlooked factor in dating. Being in tune with one's own body and emotions can lead to better understanding and empathy towards others. For men, this means being able to recognize and respond to the signals and signs of interest from potential partners more effectively. When men feel good physically, they are more likely to exude confidence, which is a key attraction factor. This confidence can be the difference between successfully engaging with a woman who may be interested and missing out on a potential connection due to insecurities or anxieties related to physical appearance.

In the realm of online dating, where profiles can sometimes be misleading, physical well-being becomes even more crucial. Red flags can often arise in profiles that may indicate a lack of care for one's health or lifestyle choices that could be detrimental in a relationship. By prioritizing their own physical health, men can better navigate these red flags, ensuring that they seek partners who share similar values in maintaining wellness. Additionally, being physically fit can empower men to set healthy boundaries in dating, fostering mutual respect and understanding in their interactions.

Ultimately, prioritizing physical well-being is not just about enhancing one's dating prospects but also about fostering a deeper connection with oneself. Men who invest time and energy into their health can cultivate a sense of fulfillment and happiness that resonates in all aspects of their lives. This self-awareness and contentment can significantly improve their dating experiences, allowing them to attract partners who appreciate and reciprocate these values. As men embark on their dating journeys, recognizing the importance of physical well-being can lead to more meaningful relationships grounded in respect, attraction, and emotional health.

Chapter 8: Exploring the Benefits of Being Single vs. Being in a Relationship

The Advantages of Being Single

The journey of navigating the complexities of modern dating can often lead men to question the merits of singlehood versus the pursuit of a romantic relationship. In the context of understanding women's signals and signs of interest, it is essential to recognize the distinct advantages of being single. Embracing this phase can foster personal growth, enhance emotional well-being, and ultimately prepare men for more fulfilling connections when they choose to enter the dating scene.

One of the primary advantages of being single is the opportunity for self-discovery. This period allows men to explore their interests, passions, and goals without the influence or expectations of a partner. Singlehood provides the freedom to travel, engage in hobbies, and invest in personal development. By focusing on oneself, men can cultivate a deeper understanding of their values and aspirations, which is crucial when evaluating potential partners in the future. This self-awareness not only leads to more satisfying relationships but also empowers men to establish healthier dynamics when the time comes.

In addition to personal growth, being single can significantly enhance emotional resilience. Men often face societal pressures to pursue relationships, sometimes leading to hasty decisions driven by fear of loneliness. However, embracing singlehood allows individuals to build self-sufficiency and emotional stability. This strength will serve them well in future relationships, as they will be better equipped to establish healthy boundaries and communicate their needs effectively. Emotional health is a vital consideration in partner selection, and the time spent being single can fortify men against the pitfalls of unhealthy attachments.

Another significant advantage is the ability to cultivate a robust social network. Being single often provides the freedom to deepen friendships and forge new connections without the constraints of a romantic relationship. Engaging with friends and family can create a strong support system that enhances overall life satisfaction. This social capital is invaluable; it not only enriches one's life experience but also offers insights into the dynamics of relationships. Through diverse interactions, men can gain perspective on what they seek in a partner and what behaviors may be red flags in potential relationships.

Finally, the single life presents the unique opportunity to explore dating without the pressures of commitment. This exploration can be particularly enlightening, allowing men to experience various interactions and learn how to recognize genuine signs of interest from women. By navigating this phase with an open mind, men can better understand the intricacies of attraction and connection, ultimately leading to more meaningful encounters. The lessons learned during this time can be instrumental in preparing for a serious relationship when the right person comes along.

In conclusion, while society often emphasizes the importance of being in a relationship, the advantages of being single are profound and multifaceted. From fostering self-discovery and emotional resilience to enhancing social connections and dating experiences, this period can be a time of invaluable growth. For men of any age, recognizing and embracing the benefits of singlehood can pave the way for healthier, more fulfilling relationships in the future. Instead of viewing single life as a phase to escape, it can be seen as a critical step toward a deeper understanding of oneself and what one truly desires in a partner.

The Value of Healthy Relationships

In the journey of dating and relationships, the significance of healthy connections cannot be overstated. Healthy relationships serve as a foundation not only for romantic partnerships but also for personal growth and emotional well-being. Men of all ages navigating the complexities of modern dating, whether online or offline, must prioritize the value of cultivating relationships that foster mutual respect, trust, and emotional support. Recognizing the characteristics of a healthy relationship can empower men to make informed choices, avoiding pitfalls that may arise from unhealthy dynamics.

Understanding the dynamics of healthy relationships involves recognizing the importance of open communication and mutual understanding. Effective communication allows partners to express their thoughts, feelings, and needs candidly, paving the way for deeper emotional connections. This is particularly crucial in online dating, where misinterpretations can lead to misunderstandings and potential scams. By fostering a culture of transparency, men can better gauge a partner's genuine interest and intentions, reducing the risk of falling prey to manipulative behaviors often associated with online dating scams.

Moreover, healthy relationships emphasize the necessity of establishing boundaries. In the context of modern dating, where personal space and emotional availability can sometimes blur, setting clear boundaries is essential for maintaining respect and individuality. Men must recognize that boundaries are not merely restrictions but are guidelines that enhance mutual respect and understanding. This is particularly relevant when considering age differences in relationships, as varying life experiences and perspectives can influence how boundaries are perceived and respected. By engaging in discussions about boundaries early on, men can cultivate relationships that honor both partners' needs.

The emotional and physical health considerations in partner selection play a critical role in building lasting relationships. A partner's emotional intelligence, resilience, and ability to navigate life's challenges can significantly impact the overall health of a relationship. Men should reflect on their own emotional health and how it aligns with potential partners. This self-awareness not only assists in recognizing signs of interest but also ensures that both partners contribute positively to each other's well-being. By focusing on emotional and physical compatibility, men can make choices that lead to fulfilling, supportive partnerships.

Ultimately, healthy relationships provide a sense of belonging and fulfillment that enriches one's life experience. They offer a refuge from the stresses of daily life and serve as a source of encouragement and motivation. While the allure of being single can be appealing, the benefits of being in a healthy relationship—such as shared experiences, emotional support, and personal growth—are invaluable. Men should strive to find partners who not only ignite their interest but also align with their values and aspirations, allowing both individuals to thrive together. By prioritizing healthy relationships, men can navigate the intricate landscape of dating with confidence and clarity.

Making Informed Choices

Making informed choices in the realm of dating is essential for men of all ages, especially in a landscape that is increasingly complex and nuanced. The modern dating scene is rife with opportunities but also fraught with potential pitfalls, including online scams, unhealthy relationships, and cultural misunderstandings. Understanding how to navigate these challenges requires a discerning eye and a willingness to engage critically with the signals and signs presented by potential partners. This subchapter aims to empower men to make choices that not only enhance their dating experiences but also promote emotional and physical well-being.

One of the foremost considerations in making informed choices is the recognition of red flags, particularly in online dating. The rise of digital platforms has opened doors to countless romantic possibilities, yet it has also given rise to various scams. Men should be vigilant about inconsistencies in communication, requests for money, or overly personal inquiries from individuals they have just met online. Awareness of these red flags is crucial; it serves as a protective measure against emotional manipulation and financial exploitation, ensuring that men can engage with sincerity and authenticity.

Age differences in relationships can also present unique challenges and benefits. While some may view age as merely a number, it often carries implications regarding life experience, maturity, and future goals. Men should engage in open conversations about these differences, fostering understanding and respect for each other's perspectives. Making informed choices in this area requires a willingness to reflect on one's own values and what is non-negotiable in a partner. This self-awareness can lead to healthier relationships that are built on a solid foundation of mutual respect and shared life goals.

Building healthy boundaries is another critical aspect of navigating modern dating. Men must recognize that establishing boundaries is not only a sign of self-respect but also fosters a respectful dynamic in any relationship. Clear communication about personal limits, expectations, and emotional needs can prevent misunderstandings and resentment. It is essential to approach boundary-setting with empathy and openness, allowing for a dialogue that respects both partners' comfort levels. This practice not only strengthens the relationship but also enhances personal growth and emotional resilience.

Finally, understanding the emotional and physical health considerations in partner selection cannot be overstated. Men should prioritize partners who align with their mental and emotional well-being, recognizing that a healthy relationship is built on mutual support and understanding. This includes being aware of one's own emotional needs and recognizing the signs of interest from a potential partner. By honing this awareness, men can create connections that are not only rewarding but also conducive to personal growth. Ultimately, making informed choices in dating requires a balanced approach that values self-awareness, communication, and respect for oneself and others, paving the way for fulfilling and meaningful relationships.

Chapter 9: International Dating: Cultural Differences and Relationship Dynamics

Understanding Cultural Nuances

Understanding cultural nuances is paramount for men navigating the complex landscape of modern dating, especially in a world where online interactions frequently bridge geographic and cultural divides. Each culture carries its own set of values, beliefs, and communication styles, which profoundly influence how individuals express interest and affection. For men seeking to decode the signals of potential partners, recognizing these cultural differences can be the key to understanding whether a woman is genuinely interested or simply adhering to the norms of her cultural upbringing.

In many cultures, direct communication is valued, while in others, indirect signals may be more common. For instance, in Western societies, expressions of interest might be overt and straightforward, with individuals openly discussing their feelings and intentions. Conversely, in some Eastern cultures, subtlety and nuance dominate interactions, and a woman's interest may be conveyed through body language, context, or even through third parties. Men must develop an awareness of these cultural subtleties to avoid misinterpretation and to respond appropriately to the signals they receive. This understanding not only aids in building rapport but also fosters respect for the cultural background of the woman in question.

The impact of age differences in relationships can be further complicated by cultural expectations. In some cultures, older men dating younger women may be seen as socially acceptable, while in others, it could be viewed with skepticism or disapproval. Such societal norms can influence how both partners perceive their roles within the relationship, affecting dynamics such as communication styles, expectations, and emotional expressions. Men must navigate these dynamics with sensitivity, ensuring they respect cultural traditions while also establishing a mutually enjoyable relationship that honors both partners' values.

Building healthy boundaries in modern dating is another area where cultural nuances play a critical role. Different cultures have varying perspectives on dating practices, personal space, and emotional intimacy. For example, some cultures may emphasize a slower, more cautious approach to physical intimacy, while others may adopt a more liberal attitude. Men should be attentive to these boundaries, recognizing that what may be acceptable in one cultural context might be inappropriate in another. Establishing clear communication about boundaries can help bridge these gaps and ensure that both partners feel comfortable and respected throughout their dating journey.

Lastly, international dating requires a keen understanding of how cultural differences can influence relationship dynamics, including the way interest is expressed and reciprocated. Men must be prepared to adapt their approaches based on their partner's cultural background, whether that involves altering their communication style, being mindful of differing expectations, or understanding the significance of family involvement in relationships. By embracing cultural nuances and demonstrating respect for their partner's heritage, men can cultivate deeper connections that transcend cultural barriers, ultimately leading to more fulfilling and meaningful relationships.

Communication Across Cultures

Effective communication is a cornerstone of any successful relationship, yet it becomes even more crucial in the context of cross-cultural interactions. As men navigate the complex waters of modern dating, especially in an increasingly globalized world, understanding the nuances of communication across cultures can significantly impact their dating experiences.

Different cultures come with varying norms, values, and expectations, all of which influence how individuals express interest, affection, and intent. For men seeking to decode the signals and signs of interest from women from diverse backgrounds, awareness of these cultural differences is essential.

Language barriers are often the most apparent challenge in cross-cultural communication. The subtleties of tone, body language, and even silence can convey entirely different meanings depending on one's cultural upbringing. For instance, direct eye contact may be seen as a sign of confidence and engagement in some cultures, while in others, it might be interpreted as disrespect or aggression. Men should be attuned to these variations, recognizing that what may seem like a lack of interest could simply be an unfamiliarity with the more overt expressions commonly found in their own culture. Developing a keen sensitivity to these differences can help men read the signs of interest more accurately and respond appropriately.

Additionally, cultural expectations around dating can significantly influence how relationships develop. In some cultures, traditional gender roles may dictate that men take the lead in initiating romantic encounters, while in others, women may be more empowered to express their interest openly. Understanding these dynamics is crucial for men who wish to navigate online dating scams and recognize red flags. By being aware of cultural norms, they can better assess whether a woman's behavior aligns with her cultural background or if it raises concerns about authenticity or underlying motives.

The impact of age differences in relationships can also be shaped by cultural perspectives. In certain cultures, significant age gaps may be more acceptable, while in others, they can lead to misunderstandings and social stigma. For men, particularly those engaging with international dating, it is vital to approach these age-related dynamics with an open mind. Recognizing that perceptions of maturity, stability, and relationship suitability can vary widely across cultures can help men find the right balance in their interactions. This understanding fosters healthy boundaries and promotes respect for individual preferences and cultural backgrounds.

Finally, the journey of dating across cultures is enriched by personal stories and experiences. Men who actively seek to learn from both their successes and failures in cross-cultural relationships can gain invaluable insights. Sharing these experiences not only helps in personal growth but also builds a sense of community among those navigating similar challenges. As men strive to understand emotional connections and the intricacies of international dating, they must remain adaptable and empathetic, appreciating the beauty of cultural diversity while honing their ability to decode women's signals and signs of interest.

Building Bridges in Diverse Relationships

Building bridges in diverse relationships requires a nuanced understanding of the unique dynamics that accompany varying backgrounds, experiences, and expectations. In today's dating landscape, where interactions often transcend cultural, age, and lifestyle differences, establishing meaningful connections demands both awareness and adaptability. For men navigating these multifaceted relationships, recognizing the signals of interest while being attuned to the potential complexities can significantly enhance the quality of their interactions.

One of the most critical aspects of building bridges in diverse relationships is effective communication. Misunderstandings can easily arise when partners come from different cultural or social backgrounds. It is essential to cultivate an open dialogue that allows both individuals to express their thoughts, feelings, and concerns. This is especially true in online dating, where profiles may not fully represent a person's values or intentions. Men should be proactive in asking clarifying questions and sharing their perspectives, ensuring that both parties feel heard and understood. This foundational step not only mitigates potential miscommunications but also fosters trust and intimacy.

Age differences in relationships can present both challenges and opportunities. Men may find themselves drawn to partners significantly younger or older, each bringing unique life experiences that shape their expectations and desires. It is vital to approach these differences with respect and curiosity rather than judgment. Engaging in discussions about life goals, values, and relationship aspirations can help bridge the generational gap. Such conversations can lead to a deeper understanding of one another's perspectives, allowing both partners to navigate their relationship dynamics with empathy and consideration.

Establishing healthy boundaries is another essential component of building bridges in diverse relationships. In the modern dating environment, where interactions can often become overwhelming or ambiguous, clearly defined boundaries serve as a guiding framework. Men should strive to communicate their needs and limits while remaining open to their partner's expectations. This practice not only protects individual well-being but also shapes a relationship environment where both parties feel safe and respected. Healthy boundaries can help mitigate feelings of resentment or misunderstanding, paving the way for a more balanced and fulfilling connection.

Ultimately, the journey of building bridges in diverse relationships is enriched by mutual respect, open communication, and a willingness to learn from one another. By recognizing the unique aspects of their partner's background and experiences, men can foster genuine connections that transcend superficial attraction. Embracing diversity as a strength rather than a challenge can lead to profound personal growth and satisfaction in relationships. As men reflect on their dating experiences, they should remain mindful that every interaction holds the potential for deeper understanding, connection, and love.

Chapter 10: Personal Stories of Dating Success and Failure: Lessons Learned

Inspiring Success Stories

In the realm of dating, success stories often serve as a beacon of hope and inspiration for men navigating the complex landscape of romantic relationships. These narratives not only highlight the potential for meaningful connections but also emphasize the importance of understanding and interpreting the signals and signs of interest from women. By reflecting on real-life experiences, men can gain valuable insights into the dynamics of attraction and the nuances that differentiate a fleeting encounter from a lasting relationship.

One inspiring success story comes from a man in his mid-thirties who, after years of unsuccessful online dating, decided to take a step back and reassess his approach. He realized that he had been too focused on finding immediate connections rather than fostering genuine relationships. By shifting his mindset and prioritizing healthy boundaries, he began to engage with women on a more authentic level. This approach not only helped him recognize signs of interest more clearly but also allowed him to create a dating environment where both parties felt respected and valued. Ultimately, he found a partner who matched his values and aspirations, illustrating the importance of self-reflection and patience in the dating process.

Another powerful narrative involves a man in his fifties who found love with a woman significantly younger than himself. Initially apprehensive about the age difference, he learned to embrace it by focusing on shared interests and mutual respect rather than societal expectations. Through open communication and an understanding of each other's perspectives, they built a relationship that thrived on emotional connection and compatibility. This story highlights how age differences can be navigated successfully when both partners are willing to engage in honest conversations and prioritize each other's needs, reinforcing that love knows no boundaries when approached with maturity and understanding.

Personal stories of overcoming online dating scams also provide valuable lessons. A man in his late twenties encountered a fraudulent profile that initially captivated him with charm and charisma. However, he recognized red flags early on, such as inconsistencies in communication and evasiveness about personal details. By trusting his instincts and conducting thorough research, he was able to extricate himself from a potentially harmful situation. This experience reinforced the importance of vigilance and skepticism in online dating, while also illustrating that awareness and education can empower men to protect themselves from deceitful encounters.

In a world where dating norms continue to evolve, the success stories of those who have navigated the complexities of modern relationships serve as a reminder that understanding and empathy are key components of any romantic connection. Whether dealing with age differences, recognizing signs of interest, or establishing healthy boundaries, these narratives inspire men to approach dating with confidence and clarity. By learning from the experiences of others, men can cultivate the resilience needed to forge authentic connections and ultimately find love that is not only fulfilling but also enriching.

Cautionary Tales of Failure

In the realm of dating, particularly in a landscape dominated by online interactions and varying relationship dynamics, cautionary tales of failure serve as critical lessons for men navigating these waters. The complexities of modern dating—exacerbated by online scams, age differences, and the presence of children from previous relationships—can lead to pitfalls that may not only hurt emotionally but also impact one's financial stability and personal well-being. Understanding and recognizing these cautionary tales can empower men to make informed decisions and avoid common missteps in their quest for companionship.

Online dating platforms, while offering significant opportunities to meet potential partners, are rife with scams designed to exploit vulnerable users. Men need to be vigilant against red flags such as overly generic profiles, requests for money, or swift declarations of love from someone they have just met online. These cautionary tales often highlight individuals who, seduced by the allure of romance, found themselves victims of elaborate schemes. Learning to identify these indicators not only protects one's financial interests but also preserves emotional health, enabling men to focus on genuine connections rather than fleeting illusions.

Age differences in relationships can also pose unique challenges that may lead to failure if not navigated carefully. While love knows no age, the implications of generational gaps can affect interests, lifestyle choices, and future aspirations. Cautionary tales abound of men who, captivated by younger partners, found themselves at odds with differing life stages and expectations. Understanding how to find the right balance in age-diverse relationships is essential; mutual respect and open communication are key to fostering a healthy dynamic that precludes the common pitfalls associated with significant age gaps.

Establishing healthy boundaries is crucial in modern dating, yet many men fail to recognize their importance until it is too late. Boundaries protect emotional health and foster respect within relationships. Tales of men who neglected to set limits often reveal a cycle of dependency or resentment, leading to toxic interactions and heartbreak. Learning from these experiences emphasizes the need for self-awareness and assertiveness in expressing one's needs and desires, ultimately leading to healthier relationships where both parties feel valued and secure.

Lastly, the emotional and physical health considerations in partner selection cannot be overlooked. Men may sometimes find themselves in relationships that challenge their well-being, either through emotional turmoil or unhealthy dynamics. Cautionary tales illustrate the consequences of ignoring these aspects, with many recounting how their mental health deteriorated while trying to maintain a partnership that lacked mutual support. Realizing that love cannot be forced is essential; understanding emotional connections and the importance of compatibility in health can guide men towards relationships that enhance rather than diminish their overall well-being. By learning from these cautionary tales, men can foster a more fulfilling dating experience marked by connection, respect, and mutual growth.

Key Takeaways from Real Experiences

In the complex landscape of modern dating, men often find themselves navigating a myriad of signals and signs that indicate a woman's interest. To effectively decode these signals, it is essential to draw insights from real experiences shared by others. Such anecdotes reveal common patterns and scenarios that can illuminate the often murky waters of romantic interactions. Whether it's the subtle cues in body language or the more explicit verbal affirmations, understanding these nuances can significantly enhance a man's ability to discern genuine interest from mere friendliness.

One critical takeaway from various experiences is the importance of context in interpreting signals. For instance, a woman may exhibit signs of interest in one setting, such as a social gathering, yet behave more reservedly in a professional environment. Recognizing the impact of context allows men to approach interactions with greater sensitivity and awareness. Additionally, age differences can play a pivotal role; younger women may express interest differently than their older counterparts. Men should consider these variations when assessing signals, as what may be a clear indication of interest in one demographic could be misconstrued in another.

Establishing healthy boundaries is another vital lesson gleaned from real-life dating experiences. Many men recount situations where they misread signals due to a lack of clarity in their own boundaries or those of the woman involved. Healthy boundaries foster mutual respect and create an environment where both parties feel comfortable expressing their intentions. Stories of successful relationships often highlight how clear communication regarding boundaries can prevent misunderstandings and promote a more genuine connection.

Moreover, personal accounts reveal the significance of emotional and physical health in partner selection. Men often share experiences where they overlooked red flags, such as unresolved emotional issues or lifestyle choices, only to face challenges later in the relationship. These stories underline the necessity of assessing not just the signs of interest but also the overall well-being of a prospective partner. Prioritizing emotional and physical health can lead to more fulfilling and sustainable relationships, as both partners are better equipped to support each other.

Ultimately, the narratives of those who have navigated the dating landscape offer invaluable lessons about the pros and cons of various dating scenarios, including international dating and relationships with single parents. Each experience contributes to a deeper understanding of relationship dynamics and cultural differences, emphasizing the need for adaptability and an open mind. By reflecting on these key takeaways, men can refine their approach to dating, enhancing their ability to recognize authentic interest while fostering meaningful connections.

Chapter 11: Can Love Be Forced? Understanding Emotional Connections in Relationships

The Nature of Emotional Connections

Emotional connections are at the heart of human relationships, serving as a vital component in the dynamics of romantic engagements. For men navigating the often complex landscape of dating—whether online or in person—understanding the nature of these connections is essential. Emotional bonds foster intimacy, trust, and mutual respect, which are all crucial for a healthy relationship. Recognizing how these connections form and evolve can significantly impact one's approach to dating, allowing for deeper, more meaningful interactions that transcend superficial attraction.

In the realm of online dating, where profiles can often obscure true intentions, discerning the authenticity of emotional connections becomes even more critical. Men need to be vigilant about red flags that may indicate a lack of genuine interest or, worse, manipulative behaviors. Scammers may feign emotional connections to exploit vulnerabilities. Understanding the signs of a true emotional connection—such as consistent communication, shared experiences, and a willingness to invest time and effort—can help men navigate these treacherous waters more effectively.

Age differences in relationships can also influence the development of emotional connections. While age can bring varying life experiences and perspectives, it can also introduce challenges in emotional compatibility. Men must evaluate whether their own emotional maturity aligns with that of their partner, as this alignment is essential for nurturing a healthy bond. Differences in life stages, priorities, and expectations can complicate emotional intimacy, making it vital to engage in open conversations about these dynamics to build a strong foundation.

Healthy boundaries play a significant role in shaping emotional connections. For men, establishing and respecting boundaries is crucial for fostering a safe environment where both partners feel valued and understood. Clear communication about personal limits not only protects individual well-being but also enhances emotional intimacy. When both partners feel secure, they are more likely to share their vulnerabilities, which can deepen their connection and lead to a more fulfilling relationship.

Lastly, understanding that emotional connections cannot be forced is key to genuine relationship development. While attraction can spark initial interest, true emotional bonds take time to cultivate. Men should be attentive to the organic progression of their relationships, allowing feelings to develop naturally rather than rushing the process. By embracing patience and focusing on mutual growth, men can create strong emotional ties that form the backbone of lasting relationships, ultimately leading to a more rewarding dating experience.

The Myths of Forcing Love

The notion of forcing love is steeped in myths that can mislead men in their pursuit of genuine connections. Many believe that love is something that can be manufactured through persistence, manipulation, or even grand gestures. This misconception not only distorts the reality of emotional connections but also fosters unhealthy dynamics in relationships.

Men should be aware that love is not a commodity to be bargained for; it is an organic experience that flourishes in an environment of mutual respect and genuine interest.

One prevalent myth is the idea that persistence will eventually win over a reluctant partner. While determination can sometimes be admirable, it risks crossing the line into harassment when the other party is not reciprocating interest. Forcing a relationship can create significant emotional strain, leading to resentment rather than the desired affection. It's essential to recognize the difference between showing interest and disregarding boundaries. Understanding and respecting these boundaries is crucial for fostering a healthy relationship, where both partners feel valued and appreciated.

Another misconception is that love can be cultivated through shared experiences or by creating an idealized version of oneself. While common interests and compatibility play a significant role in attraction, they cannot substitute for genuine emotional chemistry. Men often fall into the trap of believing that if they can impress or entertain a woman enough, she will inevitably develop feelings for them. This approach can lead to superficial relationships based on performance rather than authentic connection. It is vital to focus on being oneself and allowing relationships to unfold naturally, which leads to more meaningful interactions.

Additionally, the myth that love can be forced often intersects with the idea of age differences in relationships. Many men may feel pressured to maintain a facade of maturity or stability to attract younger partners, which can result in inauthentic connections. This pressure can create imbalances in relationships, as one partner may feel compelled to adapt to the other's expectations rather than fostering an environment of equality. Recognizing that emotional maturity and compatibility matter more than age can help men navigate these dynamics more effectively, leading to healthier and more satisfying relationships.

Ultimately, the idea that love can be forced undermines the core of what relationships should be about: mutual attraction, respect, and emotional connection. Men should be encouraged to embrace vulnerability and authenticity in their dating lives, allowing love to develop naturally rather than attempting to manufacture it. By debunking these myths, they can focus on building genuine connections that stand the test of time, leading to fulfilling relationships grounded in mutual understanding and respect.

Nurturing Genuine Relationships

Nurturing genuine relationships is a vital aspect of modern dating, providing a foundation for meaningful connections that transcend the superficial. For men navigating the complexities of romantic interactions, understanding how to cultivate authentic relationships can markedly enhance their dating experiences. This involves not only recognizing the signs of interest in potential partners but also committing to open communication and emotional honesty. In an era where digital interactions often take precedence over face-to-face engagements, the challenge lies in fostering connections that are both sincere and resilient.

At the core of nurturing genuine relationships is the principle of active listening. Men should endeavor to listen attentively to their partners, demonstrating that their thoughts and feelings are valued. This goes beyond simply hearing words; it involves engaging with the message behind those words, acknowledging emotions, and responding thoughtfully. By creating an environment where open dialogue is encouraged, men can build trust and rapport, essential components of any lasting relationship. This skill becomes even more crucial in online dating scenarios, where miscommunication can easily lead to misunderstandings and, in some cases, falling victim to scams.

Establishing healthy boundaries is another critical factor in nurturing authentic relationships. Men must be clear about their own needs and limits while also respecting those of their partners. This balance fosters mutual respect and understanding, which are key to sustaining long-term connections. In today's fast-paced dating landscape, it is not uncommon for individuals to rush into relationships without adequately considering personal boundaries. Taking the time to discuss expectations and limitations can prevent potential conflicts and ensure both partners feel secure and valued.

Age differences in relationships can also play a significant role in the dynamics of genuine connections. Men should approach these situations with sensitivity, recognizing that varying life experiences can influence perspectives and priorities. Understanding and engaging with these differences can enhance the relationship, allowing both partners to learn from each other. It is essential to cultivate patience and empathy, which can bridge generational divides and create a deeper emotional connection. By doing so, men can create an atmosphere where both partners feel comfortable expressing their thoughts and desires.

Finally, recognizing the signs of interest and emotional availability is crucial in nurturing genuine relationships. Men should be attuned to both verbal and non-verbal cues from their partners, as these can provide valuable insights into their feelings. Authentic connections thrive when both individuals feel comfortable being vulnerable and expressing their true selves. By fostering an environment where emotional connections can flourish, men not only enhance their romantic prospects but also contribute to their overall personal growth. In this way, nurturing genuine relationships becomes an enriching journey that offers both partners the opportunity to evolve together, ultimately leading to more fulfilling and lasting connections.